A Consumer´s Guide to Understanding QEEG Brain Mapping and Neurofeedback Training

A Consumer´s Guide to Understanding QEEG Brain Mapping and Neurofeedback Training

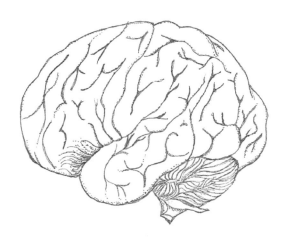

ROBERT E. LONGO, MRC, LPC, BCN

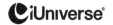

A CONSUMER'S GUIDE TO UNDERSTANDING QEEG BRAIN MAPPING AND NEUROFEEDBACK TRAINING

iUniverse books may be ordered through booksellers or by contacting:

iUniverse
1663 Liberty Drive
Bloomington, IN 47403
www.iuniverse.com
1-800-Authors (1-800-288-4677)

Because of the dynamic nature of the Internet, any web addresses or links contained in this book may have changed since publication and may no longer be valid. The views expressed in this work are solely those of the author and do not necessarily reflect the views of the publisher, and the publisher hereby disclaims any responsibility for them.

ISBN: 978-1-5320-4731-2 (sc)
ISBN: 978-1-5320-4732-9 (e)

Library of Congress Control Number: 2018904468

Print information available on the last page.

iUniverse rev. date: 05/01/2018

Contents

Preface vii

Dedication xi

Introduction.. xiii

Chapter 1   What is Quantitative
Electroencephalography (QEEG) Brain
Mapping?... 1

Chapter 2   Preparation for a QEEG—Things You
Should Know Before You Start 10

Chapter 3   Preparing for Neurofeedback 16

Chapter 4   Frequently Asked Questions (FAQs) About
Neurofeedback...21

Chapter 5   How to Optimize Your Neurofeedback
Program... 33

Appendices 41

   Appendix 1 41

   Appendix 2 45

   Appendix 3 53

   Appendix 4 55

   Appendix 5 57

   Appendix 6 61

   Appendix 7 65

   Appendix 8 69

Recommended Reading 71

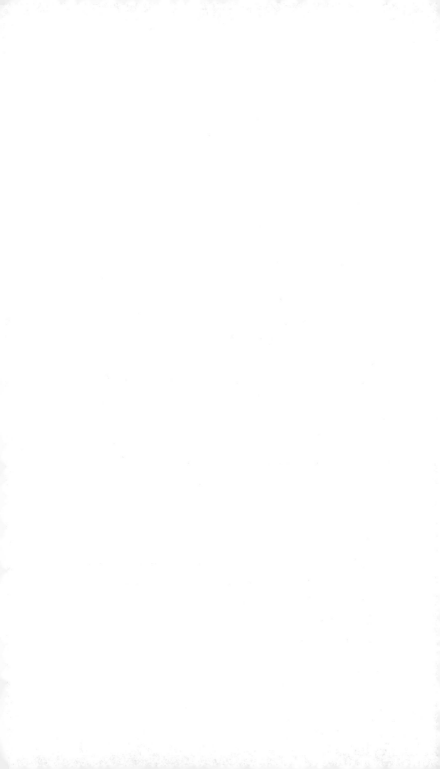

PREFACE

This booklet is specifically written for the consumer. If you are considering participating in neurofeedback, or a parent of a child, a relative, a colleague, or friend who is looking to participate in neurofeedback brain wave training, this booklet is designed to inform you about the process of being assessed for and participating in neurofeedback.

Neurofeedback is often referred to as *EEG biofeedback, neurotherapy, neurobiofeedback, and brain wave training.* These terms are generally used interchangeably, and the public often considers neurofeedback as a form of treatment or therapy. In general, I prefer to use the phrase neurofeedback *training* because providers are in fact training brainwaves to respond to the individual's unique brainwave activity via brainwave biofeedback.

In this booklet, I will cover the very basics of what I believe the reader needs to know and understand regarding neurofeedback. What is neurofeedback? How is a person assessed for participating in neurofeedback? What are the benefits? What if any are the side effects? How does one know it is helping? Does it require lifestyle changes? How long do the benefits last? What happens if it does not help? And, many more such questions and issues are addressed.

I decided to write this booklet because so many people who are interested in neurofeedback have never heard about it or do not understand what it does. Each week, new clients walk through the doors of programs and clinics throughout the United States and other countries because someone suggested that they try neurofeedback. Many new clients never knew about neurofeedback before being referred; and many mental health and health care professionals have not heard about neurofeedback.

I describe the various aspects of assessment for, preparation for, and participation in neurofeedback training. In addition, I address issues related to each of these topics including terms and definitions most commonly used by professionals who provide QEEG brain mapping and neurofeedback services. In addition, many neurofeedback providers work in conjunction with various health care professions that may include, but are not limited to, mental health professionals, medical professionals, nutritionists, social workers, and other complementary health care services.

In our respective practices, neurofeedback professionals often provide free consultation to individuals and families interested in neurofeedback training. Therefore, I am writing this booklet to parallel the information I would provide in a consultation and much more.

Finally, I am attempting to keep the information brief and easy to understand. Therefore, at the end of this booklet I have included appendices that include information about specific areas related to improving the beneficial effects of neurofeedback training, i.e., proper diet, sleep hygiene, and *examples* of the types of forms that individual practitioners may ask you to sign.

DEDICATION

In memory and tribute to a dear friend,
scholar and advocate for neurofeedback as
a means to promoting holistic wellness

Jane E. Myers, Ph.D., LPC, BCN

INTRODUCTION

Neurofeedback Training: What It Is and What It Is Not

Neurofeedback training is science's response to head injuries, life stress consequences, and a variety of conditions regulated by brain wave function. Quantitative electroencephalography (QEEG), also referred to as "brain mapping" as well as neurofeedback training are over 50 years old. Yet they are still considered new fields in many respects. A variety of innovators and professionals from diverse fields have come together to contribute their expertise to the growth of both areas. As a result, QEEG and neurofeedback enjoy a distinct and unique history.[1]

To truly understand these fields is to study the several theories regarding what neurofeedback does for the brain, the disorders it helps, and the best way to employ it. Each theory has its advocates. Thus, responsible practitioners avoid making claims of curing a disorder but instead offer explanations of how symptoms can be moderated through brainwave training and lifestyle considerations (e.g., diet,

---

[1] Soutar, R., & Longo, R.E. (2011). Doing Neurofeedback.: An Introduction. San Rafael, CA: ISNR Research Foundation.

sleep habits). Additionally, the length of treatment (brain wave training) varies among clients. Effective neurofeedback usually takes 30–40 sessions on average. Some clients, however, attain results within 20 sessions while others may require more than 60 sessions for treatment to be effective. When clients reach their goals for symptom relief, enhanced quality of daily life, etc., an additional 5–10 sessions are often conducted to help consolidate the benefits of neurofeedback training.[2]

Neurofeedback is an intervention used to improve, or if you will address or treat, disorders of the brain and the central nervous system. Some of the more common disorders and symptoms include anxiety, depression, insomnia cognitive deficits, focus and concentration deficits, emotional deficits, headaches, pain, among other problems. Neurofeedback's history dates back over 50 years and was initially used to treat seizures, attention deficit, and addictions. Neurofeedback is generally considered to be safe and non-intrusive; and generally, does not produce harmful side effects.

---

[2] Soutar, R., & Longo, R.E. (2011). Doing Neurofeedback.: An Introduction. San Rafael, CA: ISNR Research Foundation.

CHAPTER ONE

What is Quantitative Electroencephalography (QEEG) Brain Mapping?

Quantitative EEG (QEEG) is a set or group of numerical and statistical methods used to analyze and assess a properly acquired EEG (brain waves). It is used to learn how your brain supports the activities you do. It is not used to make medical diagnoses and is different from medical procedures like CT scans, fMRI, SPECT and PET. QEEG measures the various brain waves and their activity in the lobes of the brain. In most cases a full QEEG collects information at 19 locations on the scalp of the head referred to as the 10-20 International System. Thus, a QEEG produces measures for each of the 10-20 scalp locations. It will describe the amount or power for each brainwave frequency or group of frequencies called bands. QEEG also determines how brainwaves at one location relate to those at another location providing measures for similarity in power, speed and consistency of communication. In order to determine whether your measures are likely to be associated with your concerns, your measures are compared to one or more *databases*. Most databases compare your EEG measurements to those of a large number of so-called "normal" people to see if you are statistically different from them. Other databases compare your EEG to groups of people with a certain disorder, to see if you are statistically similar to them.

QEEG has become more standardized but there are still several techniques, models, and methods used to gather QEEG data. At this time, QEEG is not considered a stand-alone diagnostic tool; therefore, it is typically used in conjunction with other diagnostic procedures and testing. However, QEEG can help support established or suspected diagnoses. Therefore, it has a differential diagnosis value. Periodic QEEG retesting clients once neurofeedback has begun helps to provide evidence for neurofeedback practitioners that neurofeedback is having the desired effect.[3]

There are four lobes of the brain, the frontal Lobes, the temporal lobes, the parietal lobes, and the occipital lobes. The lobes of the brain (see Figure 1) are collectively referred to as the cortex. In addition, there are two specialized areas that are referred to as the prefrontal cortex; and the motor strip and sensory motor strip (see Figure 2). If your provider reviews your brain map with you, the following information helps further explain how the map is viewed.

---

[3] Soutar, R., & Longo, R.E. (2011). Doing Neurofeedback.: An Introduction. San Rafael, CA: ISNR Research Foundation.

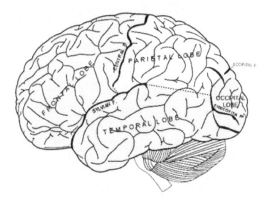

Figure 1. Left side view of the lobes of the brain.[4]

Why Get a QEEG if I Already Have Cognitive and Emotional Testing?

QEEG provides information about how your brain supports the cognitive abilities and emotions measured by other measures. In this way QEEG provides information to design a method to train your brain directly.

The brain is divided into two hemispheres, the right and left hemisphere, and the 10-20 system gathers information from each lobe which is divided into left and right. In Chapter Two, Figure 4 shows the 10-20 sites most commonly used to collect basic brain wave data. The letter in front of each site indicates the lobe of the brain from which the data are being collected and the number that follows is a precise location on the scalp. The left hemisphere sites all have odd numbers (i.e., F3, T3,

[4] Soutar, R., & Longo, R.E. (2011). Doing Neurofeedback.: An Introduction. San Rafael, CA: ISNR Research Foundation.

P3, O1) and the right hemisphere sites are all followed by an even number (i.e., F4, T4, P4, O2). The motor strip (part of the frontal lobe is noted as the letter "C." For example, C3 is the left side of the motor strip. P4 is the parietal lobe right side and O1 is the left side of the occipital lobe. Thus, F4 identifies a specific location on the right side of the frontal lobe. The very most forward section of the frontal lobes over the eyes on the forehead is referred to as the prefrontal cortex.

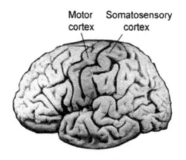

Figure 2. Left side view of the motor and somatosensory cortex. Soutar and Longo 2011

As noted above, the brain is divided into two hemispheres (see Figure 3), and the division goes right down the middle which is often referred to as the midline. In the 10-20 system, the midline is identified by the letter z (in lower case) and those sites include Fpz, Fz, Cz, Pz, and Oz (note: Fpz and Oz are generally sites that are NOT included in traditional 10-20 full QEEG measurements). In some offices and QEEG mapping systems, mini-Qs are performed and those measure only include 10 sites (F3, F4, C3, C4, T3, T4, P3, P4 and O1, O2).

The right hemisphere is slightly larger in normal adults, and is responsible for the following:

- Emotional Quotient (E.Q.)
- swearing
- early self-concept
- social encoding
- social skills
- face recognition
- emotional processes
- negative emotions
- empathy
- nonverbal expression and association
- spatial memory and problem solving
- auditory processing
- musical processing

The left hemisphere is generally responsible for the following:

- I.Q.
- logic
- verbal association
- verbal expression
- verbal memory
- auditory processing
- word recognition
- math and grammar problem solving

Left-side brain problems often correspond with a tendency toward significant irritability and even violence.

LEFT   RIGHT

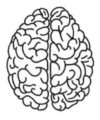

Figure 3. Right and left hemispheres of the brain.

Brainwaves

Brainwaves are basically divided into four types, *delta* waves, *theta* waves, *alpha* waves and *beta* waves which are further divided into slow beta waves and fast beta waves. These waves or bandwidths are measured in Hertz. A Hertz is a specific frequency that defines the speed of that bandwidth. In comparison, one might think about a radio. A radio has two major bands, AM and FM. Each of these bands has frequencies that go up and down a scale and to some degree organize the types of programming one might hear. For example, in the FM stations the lower numbers e.g., 88.5 might be news and/or classical music. Mid-range stations, e.g., 95.1 might be jazz, and the upper stations, e.g., 105.3 are often rock stations.

Delta waves are the slowest of the brain waves and are defined as 1–3 Hertz (Hz). They might be considered as representative of the physical health of the brain and are generated from the brain stem. Delta waves are the slowest recorded brain waves in the human brain. Delta waves are associated with deep levels of relaxation and restorative sleep.

6

They also have been found to be involved in unconscious bodily functions such as regulating heart beat and digestion. Adequate production of delta waves helps us get a good night's sleep. Abnormal delta wave activity may be indicative of learning disabilities or attention and cognitive deficits and are often indicative of traumatic brain injury (TBI).[5]

Theta waves are the next slowest wave (4–7Hz), but faster than delta and are generated from the limbic system (emotions and memory). Theta waves are sometimes referred to as getting into a day-dreamy or dissociative state. These waves play a role in our experiencing and feeling deep and raw emotions. Too much theta activity can be indicative of ADHD, hyperactivity, and impulsivity; and too little theta can be indicative of poor emotional awareness.[6]

Alpha waves also are considered a slow wave (8–12 Hz) but are faster than Theta. They are generated from the thalamus and are considered regulatory. Alpha waves constitute our being in a relaxed and calm state but ready to gear up or further calm down. Alpha is the pathway to sleep. When an individual, shifts from alpha to theta, the person "checks out" and moves into theta and more of a daydream dissociative state. When some people become stressed, "alpha blocking" may occur which involves excessive beta activity and very little alpha. Too much alpha is indicative of poor sleep, depression and anxiety. Too little alpha is indicative of stress, adrenal fatigue, confusion, reduced cognitive stamina, and cognitive processing deficits.

---

[5] http://mentalhealthdaily.com/2014/04/15/5-types-of-brain-waves-frequencies-gamma-beta-alpha-theta-delta/

[6] Ibid.

Beta waves are the fast wave of the brain and are generated from the cortex (13–30Hz). Beta waves are high frequency waves that are commonly observed while we are awake. Beta waves are involved in conscious thought, logical thinking, and information processing as when learning. They allow us to focus and complete school- or work-based tasks easily. Having too much beta may lead to us to experiencing excessive stress and/or anxiety, high arousal, and an inability to relax. If you have lower levels of beta you may have ADHD, find yourself daydreaming, feeling depressed and having poor cognitive processing.

QEEG Brain Map

When a QEEG is performed the brainwaves are measured in all four lobes at each of the 10-20 sites. The data are collected and then transformed into a pictorial representation of brain activity known as a QEEG brain map. QEEG should not be considered diagnostic. No one should perform a QEEG on you and tell you that you have a particular diagnosis, i.e., anxiety, Parkinson's, insomnia. However, QEEG is commonly and ethically used for purposes of differential diagnosis. In other words, a client or patient may say that they have been diagnosed with depression or describe a list of symptoms that often are associated with depression. When the QEEG map is completed the provider may say that the QEEG is indicative of someone who has depression based upon the clinician's knowledge and experience. Thus, QEEG interpretation is most commonly done in conjunction with other testing that might include emotional measures, cognitive measures, physical health symptoms, and a history taken from the prospective patient or client by the provider, referring clinician, or other health care provider.

Insurance

Ask your insurance provider if you have out of panel benefits. Common procedure codes that might be used are 90901 or 90876.

CHAPTER TWO

Preparation for a QEEG—Things You Should Know Before You Start

Once you have decided to pursue having a QEEG the clinician will have you or your representative fill out and sign forms, complete paperwork, take a history, and may have you take certain tests or complete questionnaires. Some of the paperwork you read, complete, and sign may include, for example: a Client's Rights and Responsibilities (see Appendix 1), Informed Consent (Appendix 2), Financial Statement (Appendix 3), Release of Information (if you want results shared with another professional; Appendix 4) and a Client Acknowledgement form (Appendix 5).

Most providers will have a similar routine for preparing the client/patient for a brain map despite different pieces of equipment. In most cases, instructions given to the client will be very similar (see Appendix 6). You will note that the process entails only passive reading of brain wave activity, i.e., the patient/client does not experience any discomfort.

Typically, a simple measure of the client's head size is taken. The forehead, earlobes and locations on the scalp are cleaned with a special cleanser. A colored nylon stretch cap with 20 electrodes (or similar device), is placed on the head. An ear-clip is placed on each ear lobe and a special conductive gel is used to fill each electrode. Once the prep procedure is completed, the provider checks the quality of readings from each electrode site, and the client/patient is then instructed about the need to quietly sit still. Movements such as jaw clenching, eye blink, frowning, and other head and facial movements are discouraged during the time QEEG measures are taken because they create artifact that results in poor readings.

The patient/client is then placed in a comfortable chair and instructed to sit up straight with both feet on the ground, arms on the chair armrests or lap, and to not cross arms, legs or ankles during the procedure. Measurements are then taken with both the patient/client's eyes closed and eyes open. Depending on equipment being used and the client's ability to relax and sit still during measurements, the process of data collection takes between 15–30 minutes.

With some equipment and QEEG mapping systems the results of the QEEG can be uploaded, automatically artifacted (a process by which poor measures generated by movement are removed), and a brain map created within a few minutes is ready for review with the patient/client. Most systems, however, require the clinician to review the raw data and edit out artifact before the data can be loaded and run to produce a map. This process can take considerable amounts of time so the results are reviewed with the patient/client at a later date.

Interpreting Results to Clients

There are a variety of neurofeedback systems available to providers that are capable of doing both QEEG assessments and neurofeedback training. These systems are more similar than different but often have slight differences in the way they gather and process EEG signals and the maps that they produce. Therefore, if two different systems (pieces of equipment) using unique software are used to gather EEG data from the same individual, the software used to show brainwaves likely will be similar in most ways but different in the depictions that they use to produce the visual aspects of QEEG assessment. The bottom line; they will be much more similar than different, yielding similar but not always the exact same results. This should not be a concern to the consumer. If you go to a provider using one piece of equipment and specific software and you then went to another provider using different equipment and software both QEEG Brain Maps will yield similar results but the maps may look different visually.

How Your QEEG Map Can Relate to Brain Wave Activity and Typical Self-Reported Conditions

As noted above, QEEG brain maps should not be used for diagnostic purposes but are useful tools for assessing the degree to which a symptom or problem exists. Each electrode site as noted above can be correlated to particular brain functions. When there is an abnormality it may show up in one or more ways and these abnormalities in turn are then compared to or matched with the client's self-reported symptom(s). Table 1 below is a partial list of Brodmann areas (parts of the brain associated with particular brain functions). The Brodmann areas as associated with specific 10-20 location sites (Figure 4). This further helps the clinician pair the client's self-reported symptoms to the QEEG findings.

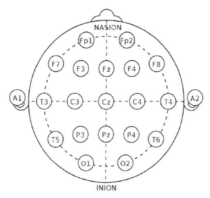

Figure 4. International 10-20 System for Electrode Placement.

Table 1

Brodmann Areas

10-20 Site	Brodmann Area	Function
Fpz	10, 11, 32	Emotional inhibition, oversensitivity, impulsivity, motivation, attention
Fz	8, 6, 9	Personality changes
Fp1	10, 11, 46	Cognitive emotional valancing, irritability, intrusiveness, depression, social awareness, positive emotion, like
Fp2	10, 11, 46	Emotional inhibition, impulsivity, tactlessness, mania, social awareness, negative emotion, dislike
F7	45, 47, 46	Working memory, divided and selective attention, filtering, word retrieval
F8	45, 47, 46	Intonation of speech, working memory, facial emotional processing, sustained attention
F3	8, 9, 46	Short-term memory, facial recognition, object processing, planning and problem solving
F4	8, 9, 46	Short-term memory, vigilance, selective and sustained attentional area
C3	3, 1, 4	Sensory and motor functions
C4	3, 1, 4	Sensory and motor functions
C3-C4	6, 8, 9	Sensorimotor, timing, movement, visual focus, and motion
Cz	6, 4, 3	Sensory and motor functions

T3	42, 22, 21	Language comprehension, verbal understanding, long-term memory, event sequencing
T4	42, 22,21	Personality—emotional tonality (anger, sadness), categorization and organization, visualization, auditory cortex
T5	39, 37, 19	Meaning construction, difficulty with arithmetic, short term memory
T6	39, 37, 19	Facial recognition, emotional content
Pz	7, 5, 19	Attentional shifting, perseverance
P3	7, 40, 19	Digit span problems, information organization problems, self-boundaries, excessive thinking
P4	7, 40, 19	Visual processing, vigilance, excessive self-concern, victim mentality, context boundaries, rumination
O1 & O2	18, 19, 17	Visual processing, procedural memory, dreaming, timing

Adapted from Soutar & Longo 2013[7]

[7] Soutar, R., & Longo, R.E. (2013). *Doing Neurofeedback.: An Introduction.* San Rafael, CA: ISNR Research Foundation.

CHAPTER THREE

Preparing for Neurofeedback

Once the clinician has reviewed the results of the QEEG brain map, he/she will then review with the patient/client the treatment plan. There are several things that should be explained.

Topics typically discussed, and questions often asked include but are not limited to:

- **Number of sessions.** The average number of sessions for neurofeedback varies based upon multiple factors including type of neurofeedback being done (for purposes of this booklet, all references to neurofeedback will be to traditional 1, 2 and 4 channel traditional neurofeedback brain wave training); the brain wave characteristics/symptoms/disorders being treated, the severity of the problem and intervening variables (discussed below) that can interfere with the efficacy of neurofeedback treatment. In general, the average number of sessions to address the more common disorders including ADD/ADHD, anxiety, depression, and insomnia is 30–40 sessions.

- **Frequency and duration of sessions.** Effective neurofeedback requires a patient/client's commitment to participate in the recommended schedule. Patients/ clients need to have sessions at least one time per week, and two sessions per week is common in many clinics. In some cases, patients/clients participate in three or more sessions per week.

- **Cost of sessions.** The cost per session is variable based upon the type of neurofeedback being done, the length of sessions, whether it is being billed to insurance, and other factors. Prices may range from as little as $50 per session to as much as $150 or more per session. National averages range from $120–$125 per session.

- **Insurance coverage.** Insurance may or may not cover neurofeedback and varies from one insurance company to another. Additionally, the same insurance company, i.e., BCBS, Aetna, UHC, Tricare, Cigna, etc., may cover neurofeedback in one state but not in another. You should ask your clinician for such information. The majority of neurofeedback providers, however, do not take insurance.

- **Side effects.** In general, neurofeedback has few adverse effects. Most such side effects are not considered to be negative or long lasting. For example, training with neurofeedback can occasionally result in response(s) that temporarily increase symptoms that are typically associated with relaxation and calming of the central nervous system such as fatigue, headaches, lightheadedness, dizziness, irritability, moodiness, weeping, insomnia, agitation, and difficulties with focus and anxiety. These reactions, if they occur, are temporary and typically only last 24–48 hours. Once patients/clients become more relaxed and aware, they tend to integrate past emotional issues and these symptoms subside. Therefore, counseling during the training process can be very beneficial for some patients/clients.

- **Progress or lack thereof.** There are three primary reasons why some people do not benefit from neurofeedback:

    a) **Physiological.** In this situation, the client has a health-related condition that counters the benefits of neurofeedback. For example, a person with serious G.I. disorder like irritable bowel syndrome or celiac may not progress as well or as rapidly as those who do not suffer from such disorders.

    b) **Social.** Clients who have significant life stressors may progress more slowly than those who do not. For example, chaotic home life (i.e., dysfunctional marriage and/or family) significant work stressors, problems at school i.e., being bullied, etc., can all detract from progressing in sessions.

    c) **Biological.** Taking multiple types of psychotropic medications (i.e., anti-depression, anti-anxiety), excessive alcohol consumption, etc.

- **Lifestyle changes.** As with any typ
  mental health problem, there are
  that need to be considered. Die₁
  exercise, and sleep hygiene are imɟ
  need to be considered. In addition, daily activitiᴜ
  and risk for receiving a head injury (i.e., playing
  contact sports) all should be addressed with the
  provider (see Appendices 7–9).
- **Who will provide sessions.** Many clinicians provide
  neurofeedback sessions directly. Others, use trained
  technicians who will provide neurofeedback services.

All the above areas should be discussed with the clinician who
will be providing you services. Before each session, there are
some things to do and not to do. It is important to not drink
stimulants such as coffee and other caffeinated beverages,
water is best. A small snack is helpful. High protein like a
handful of nuts is excellent. Avoid sugars and carbohydrates.

Depending upon the symptoms being treated and the type
of neurofeedback being used, you may be training with your
eyes closed or eyes opened. With your eyes closed you may
be listening to music and/or certain tones. With your eyes
open you may be watching a DVD, participating in a game
or engaged in a cognitive task.

Regardless of the type of neurofeedback training, it is
important that you do the following:

- Turn your cellphone on silent or turn it off. Do not
  keep your cell phone on your body. Keep it at least
  3 feet away from your body.

- Sit up straight in the chair and do not slouch down.
- Try to sit still and not move.
- Keep your arms and hands on your lap or the chair armrests.
- Do not cross your arms or legs.

CHAPTER FOUR

Frequently Asked Questions (Faqs) About Neurofeedback

How Does Neurofeedback Work?

Neurofeedback is an advanced intervention that presents the participant with real-time feedback on brainwave activity, as measured by sensors on the scalp, and typically in the form of visual or audio rewards. When brain activity changes in the direction desired by the neurofeedback protocol, a positive "reward" feedback is given to the individual. Most neurofeedback methods train brain waves to optimize neuro-electrical self-regulation.

Neurofeedback works by training up or down certain brain wave frequencies. *More efficient and effective brain waves patterns make the brain function more effectively and reduce problematic symptoms.* Over time (and usually after 5–6 sessions), clients should notice and feel differences in how they think, feel, and behave. For example, clients may notice improved sleep, feel more energy or motivation, improved concentration and focus, and/or feel more relaxed and calm. Changes in appetite, mental performance and overall mood also are common benefits as training sessions progress.

Most participants complete a minimum of 30–40 sessions to establish the changes neurofeedback makes in the brain. Each week, patients/clients are asked to complete a questionnaire that tracks the problem areas/symptoms to assess improvement through neurofeedback. In addition, individual lifestyle changes (as noted in this booklet's appendices) will help the benefits of neurofeedback take hold sooner. Conversely in the absence of following the advice given within this booklet, it may take longer to realize the benefits of neurofeedback. For example, if participants do not work on maintaining healthy lifestyles, the benefits of neurofeedback will not be optimal, and in some cases, minimal benefits may occur. Individuals participating in neurofeedback will receive maximum benefits if they understand the information and follow the basic instructions that are shared on the pages that follow.

What is the Success Rate of Neurofeedback?

Generally, the success rate with neurofeedback is over 90% in my experience with clients who follow my recommendations. Everyone is different, of course, and one's lifestyle and commitment to treatment are important. Some individuals are fast responders and others are not. Few individuals do not respond to neurofeedback training. I do not always know why some do not respond but often it is due to physical health or social stress problems. By following the guidelines your clinician recommends, you will ensure having the best chance of benefiting from neurofeedback. Many practitioners ask that you attend at least 10 sessions to have an opportunity to experience progress toward your goals. They will suggest 10 sessions because most people see improvements earlier, but some are late responders. It is reasonable to expect a 50% improvement and usually more to your most troubling problems with a full course of sessions.

What Should I Expect After the First Few Sessions?

In general, most trainees do not experience major changes after just 4–5 sessions. You may not experience anything after the first session or two. It is not uncommon, however, that you notice feeling calmer, more focused, more productive, less foggy, and having better sleep that night. You may sleep better but still not be able to really tell a difference overall. As you progress in neurofeedback, you will notice that the benefits last for more than 1 or 2 days. After 20 or more sessions, you should begin to experience the benefits lasting up to 1 week, or more.

What Should I Expect from Further Sessions?

The most common report is feeling more focused, calmer all the time, and improved sleep. Typically, symptoms become less intense, less frequent, and are of shorter duration. Emotional calm comes first, and then mental focus tends to improve later. Ideally, you will experience steady progress. Improvements may be experienced in any realm in your life where the brain plays a role.

Are There any Adverse Effects of Neurofeedback?

Adverse effects (risks) are rare, minor and short-term (see Appendix 5). The least likely response after a session is feeling fatigue, or the opposite, over-energized. Sometimes there can be a headache or some moodiness. This should dissipate within a few hours. On occasion, a very sensitive person will experience fatigue or sadness lasting into a second day, but this is not common. The length and frequency of training sessions can be adjusted as needed to moderate such responses. In general neurofeedback side effects may include the following:

a. Sleep differences—
generally improves
b. Increased energy level
c. Enhanced calmness
d. Enhanced focus
e. Improved concentration
f. Improved focus and
attention
g. Memory improvement
h. Reduced emotional
reactivity
i. Reduced ability to resist
emotions
j. Increased awareness of
dreams
k. Nightmares

l. Irritability (short-term
after a session)*
m. Headaches*
n. Anxiety*
o. Insomnia*
p. Agitation*
q. Relaxation
r. Boundary Clarification
(relationship changes, i.e.,
becoming more assertive)
s. Moodiness
t. Vivid dreams

* These side effects are rare and if experienced should be reported to the clinician immediately or at the beginning of the next session.

Additionally, it is important to note that other interventions used by patients/clients for purposes of relaxation may have adverse effects. For example, Perez-De-Albeniz, et al (2000)[8] note, clients/patients who practice Transcendental Meditation for relaxation and improved health, negative side effects may include: "relaxation-induced anxiety and panic; paradoxical increases in tension; less motivation in life; boredom; pain; impaired reality testing; confusion and disorientation; feeling 'spaced out'; depression; increased negativity; being more judgmental; feeling addicted to meditation; uncomfortable kinesthetic sensation; mild dissociation; feelings of guilt; psychosis-like symptoms; grandiosity; elation; destructive behavior; suicidal feelings; defenselessness; fear; anger; apprehension; and despair."

Will Other Treatments and the Medications I Am Currently Taking Affect my Neurofeedback Program?

Neurofeedback tends to make other treatment methods work better. It also seems to make medications work better at first. Psychoactive pharmaceuticals (those prescribed for ADD/ADHD, anxiety, depression, mood disorders, and insomnia) tend to slow the neurofeedback process down slightly. As you progress, and the underlying disorder improves, the same dosage may become too high, and side effects may increase as neurofeedback resolves a symptom, or symptoms, at the source in the brain. Therefore, it is important to keep

---

[8] Perez-De-Albeniz, Alberto and Holmes, Jeremy (2000). Meditation: Concepts, effects and uses in therapy. *International Journal of Psychotherapy,* 5(1): 49–58.

your physician/prescriber informed of your progress with the neurofeedback program so adjustments can be made, if appropriate, to your medication regimen.

If no medication adjustments are made, continuation with neurofeedback and continuing current medications and dosages should be discussed with your neurofeedback provider. As you progress with your neurofeedback and its efficacy may be negatively impacted if adjustments are not initiated.

Under What Conditions is Neurofeedback Less Effective in Achieving Optimal Results?

There are three situations for which neurofeedback is generally less effective.

1. When patients taking multiple medications for mental health disorders, such as anxiety, depression, ADHD, insomnia, etc., are not working with their health care prescriber to adjust their medications. This includes appropriately discontinuing medication in response to their progress with their neurofeedback program. In no case should a client use illicit street drugs, e.g., cocaine, marijuana, etc., as they also interfere with neurofeedback training.

2. When persons who experience ongoing stressors during most of their day, e.g., job related stress, or stressful relationships avoid addressing these stressors through mental health counseling and/or other mental health interventions.

3. When persons who have certain seriou
problems, i.e., serious GI problems, u
conditions, heavy metal toxicity, chemic
excessive copper); these problems can
sleep disturbances).

How Often Do I Need to Come?

Participating in neurofeedback is a commitment. One session per week is required. Two sessions per week is preferable. However, it is understandable that people today have complex lives, and can only commit to once a week. You should make your neurofeedback session appointments every week, 6–8 weeks out, as to constitute an established appointment. Neurofeedback is cumulative, and each session builds on the previous session. Skipping sessions slows down the overall process. Sessions usually last 45–50 minutes and are often booked on the hour. I, and many of my colleagues, reserve the right to terminate patients who are missing sessions and not committed to successful participation in neurofeedback.

How Long Does a Neurofeedback Training Program Last?

A course of neurofeedback is often 30 to 40 sessions. If you are attending sessions twice per week then the entire course of training lasts 15–20 weeks (4–5 months). In some cases when patients practice optimum self-care and holistic health, neurofeedback may be successful in 25–30 sessions.

ᴢ conditions are more severe and require more than
ل–60 sessions.

As the neurofeedback trainee approaches 20–25 neurofeedback
sessions, clinicians often recommend a repeat QEEG brain
mapping.

What is the Process for
Scheduling Appointments?

Progress is best when your clinician can see you on the same
day at the same time each week. Each of us has a circadian
rhythm (our internal body clock that tells our bodies when
to sleep, rise, eat, and regulates many of our physiological
processes), that changes throughout the day and the week.
Having neurofeedback training sessions at the same time on the
same day is best whenever possible. The following guidelines are
suggested when scheduling appointments for neurofeedback:

- **Establish a regular appointment schedule.** To
  assure that you have a weekly appointment for
  neurofeedback, it is suggested that you set up an
  established appointment on the same day(s) and
  at the same time(s) each week whenever possible.
  Some people work flexible schedules and cannot
  always be at an appointment on the same day and
  time each week. If you have difficulty scheduling
  an appointment, please let your neurofeedback
  clinician know right away.
- **Schedule your neurofeedback appointments
  6–8 weeks in advance.** Each week you should add

another appointment to your existir
keep your set appointment time(s`
can always cancel an appointment
a conflict. Most clinicians will require u.
give a 24-hour notice if you need to cancel. It is
difficult to fit patients in at the last minute as the
neurofeedback schedule often books up weeks in
advance.

- In many clinics, the 3:00 pm and 4:00 pm time
slots are usually reserved for children and adolescent
patients to accommodate school schedules and
prevent lost time during regular school hours.

How Do I Prepare for Each Neurofeedback Session?

Actual neurofeedback training sessions are generally 30 minutes long but with check-in, prep, and clean-up time sessions will be 45–50 minutes long. *Before coming to your neurofeedback session each week, please keep the following in mind:*

- Make sure you have shampooed your hair the night
before or the day of your session. Dirty hair and hair
products (especially hair dyes) affect impedance (the
quality of your brain wave readings) and can lower
the quality of your session.
- If you eat a meal or a snack within a few hours of
your session, try to eat protein and avoid processed
foods, especially those high in saturated fats and/
or carbohydrates, i.e., crackers, breads, chips, and

starches. Try to avoid sugars and caffeine. Proteins, fruits, vegetables and nuts are best.

- Drink a cup of plain water before your session.
- If you drink alcohol, you should not drink any the same day you have a neurofeedback session.

Use of Alcohol and Recreational Drugs

If you are investing the time and energy to attend neurofeedback sessions, you will progress better and quicker if you refrain from using alcohol and other recreational drugs while participating in neurofeedback. There is a reason why alcohol feels good and often calms the user down; it is a neurotoxin. Routine use of alcohol can negatively affect sleep and slow down one's overall progress while participating in neurofeedback. Marijuana and other recreational drugs also affect the brain and can negatively affect sleep and overall brain function.

Working Together with Your Clinician and Maintaining Regular Communication is Important to Support Positive Outcomes

Weekly Check-In

Your clinician needs to know how you are doing so that neurofeedback protocols can be adjusted if needed. After your first neurofeedback session, your clinician may check in and ask how you did after your first session. Even "nothing to report" is useful information. Each week you may be expected to fill out a progress tracker that has been customized for you and addresses several behavioral, emotional and cognitive areas. You may do so online or at the clinician's office prior to your appointment.

Medication Changes and Updates

After starting neurofeedback, advise your neurofeedback clinician right away if there is a change to any prescription you are currently taking for depression, anxiety, insomnia, ADD/ADHD, or any mental health related conditions, or if there is an addition of a new medicine to your regimen for these conditions.

Please provide your clinician with the updates to any of the following:

- Changes in medications;
- Dosage changes;
- Starting new medications;
- Decreasing or stopping medications;
- Changes in frequency of taking medications.

Note: Most psychotropic medications have effects on the brain and alter brain wave activity. That is the reason it is important to advise your neurofeedback specialist of medications you are taking and any changes to your medications, so they can check for changes in your EEG/brain waves. Withdrawal from medications should be supervised by your prescribing physician.

Head Injury

If you experience a head injury (no matter how major or minor) during the time you are being treated with neurofeedback, please make sure that you tell your neurofeedback clinician. If the head injury resulted in blackout, concussion, dizziness, headaches, nausea, vomiting, or similar symptoms, it is important to advise your clinician of this new injury immediately. Often neurofeedback will need to be stopped for a few months to allow the brain to heal itself naturally.

Lifestyle Changes and Events

If you are involved in life events or situations that are causing you stress, anxiety or depression, at work, at school, at home, in significant relationships, such as loss of job, loss of loved one, and/or any problems related to the quality of your life, please advise your clinician immediately.

CHAPTER FIVE

How to Optimize Your Neurofeedback Program

Neurofeedback is an effective and leading-edge intervention for a variety of disorders. To maximize the benefits of participating in neurofeedback consider following the guidelines below.

You Should Avoid or Use with Caution the Following:

Alcohol and Drugs

Alcohol is commonly used by adults for a variety of reasons from social to medicinal. Alcohol will negatively affect your sleep. On the day you have neurofeedback you should avoid any alcohol. Many practitioners will advise you to stop the use of alcohol altogether during the time you are engaged in neurofeedback training. However, I caution to limit it to occasionally (not every night) and no more than one beer or a glass of wine per day and NOT before you go to bed. Avoid hard liquor.

Recreational/Illegal Drugs

For obvious reasons, do not take any illegal substances. Alcohol, marijuana and other recreational drugs affect sleep and your brain wave activity. They too, will counter the benefits of neurofeedback. Recreational drugs such as marijuana can slow neurofeedback progress and efficacy down by 50% or more.

Neurotoxins

Aspartame is a neurotoxin (toxic to your brain) found in many diet sodas and diet foods. Neurotoxins are chemicals or additives that can directly affect the brain and nervous system.

Cosmetics

Parabens and phthalates are additives to shampoos, cosmetics and other products and can cause cancer.

Hygiene

Antiperspirants with aluminum-based compounds. Aluminum can create heavy metal toxicity.

Food Allergy and Sensitivity

Food sensitivities are present in many people and certain products such as corn, corn syrup, refined sugars, nuts, wheat, soy, dairy, are common foods to which that people have sensitivities. For example, gluten often affects the digestive system in negative ways including bloating.

Food

Processed foods are often loaded with food dyes, preservatives and other chemicals that can negatively affect your health.

Fad diets

Talk with your physician or a nutritionist before starting a new diet.

Supplements

Supplements should be taken with caution and under the guidance of your physician, a registered dietician or nutrition specialist.

Environment

Stressful environments create, maintain, and/or worsen anxiety. Try to avoid stressful situations at work and at home whenever possible. Work to find solutions to problems that minimize stress and anxiety. Often, children easily notice stress and tension in the home. Counseling may help to moderate these conditions.

Technology

Excessive time on electronics is not advised for youth with ADD and ADHD. We live in an age of technology. Many of us are using it all day long. The average child between the ages of 7–18 spends an average of 10 hours per day using electronic devices such as television, radio, computers, electronic games, cell phones, MP3 players, etc. For children under age 7 it is recommended that they not spend more than 2 hours per day in front of a screen including computer, TV, games, cell phones, etc.

Electromagnetic Waves/Fields (EMF)

Some people are sensitive to electromagnetic fields and it can affect their quality of sleep. In some cases, it can cause insomnia. Examples are electronics with remote controls, Wi-Fi computers, cellular phones, etc. If you believe you are sensitive to these waves turn everything off (unplug them) in your house before you go to sleep.

Can EMFs really affect human health? Today, over a thousand research studies have linked EMFs to important biological effects and health disorders. However, there is still great controversy about the seriousness of the health effects, and the conclusiveness of the research data. EMFs can cause interference problems for sensitive electronics and computer systems, and now, some of the research is beginning to suggest that low-level EMFs can indeed influence and interfere with sensitive bio-electromagnetic processes within our cells, brains and bodies. For example, research suggests that our pineal gland can somehow sense the daily changes of the earth's natural magnetic field and uses this information to help regulate our wake/sleep cycle. Studies indicate that artificial magnetic fields can suppress the secretion of melatonin from the pineal gland at night, the main hormone that initiates our sleep cycle.

Things to Do That Enhance your Neurofeedback Training

Routine Lifestyle

Many doctors and health professions will encourage you to try to live a routine lifestyle. What I mean by a routine lifestyle, is going to bed about the same time and getting up about the same time each day and trying to eat meals about the same time each day. This is good for both mind and body. It keeps your entire body in sync with your circadian rhythms.

It is also important to avoid situations that are known stressors whenever possible. When faced with stressful situations, work towards resolution, and try not to ruminate or "get stuck" in negative and/or destructive and nonproductive thought patterns, emotions, and destructive behaviors. When negative thoughts and emotions come up, you should talk with a professional helper. Typically, it is not helpful to keep feelings in or ignore them. Be mindful of maintaining a supportive environment at home, work, and/or school as well as a supportive peer group. Tell your clinician if you need assistance finding a reputable counseling practitioner.

Exercise

It is important to exercise 3–5 days per week. It is recommended that children and adults get the equivalent of 45 minutes of cardiovascular workout each day. If you have a sedentary job, (i.e., desk job) get up and walk around whenever possible. It is recommended that persons with lfestyles try to walk a minimum of 5000 steps

Sleep (see Appendix 7)

Most Americans do not get enough sleep! In general, children need between 8–10 hours of sleep per night and most adults, including college students, need 7–9 hours of sleep per night. Try to practice good sleep hygiene. Good sleep hygiene includes using the bedroom primarily as a place to sleep. Maintain a regular hour for going to bed. Use only incandescent lighting as all other forms of indoor lighting negatively affect the brain's bio-regulatory capacities. This pertains to daytime indoor lighting as well. Three hours before retiring dim all the lights in your environment. Use as few light sources as possible. Try to avoid watching TV when you are going to sleep. Do NOT use the computer, or any other electronic devices with a screen (i.e., iPads, cell phones, games, electronic books, etc.) at least one hour before going to sleep.

While fluorescent light bulbs and LED lights are much more energy-efficient than incandescent lights, they also tend to produce more blue light. That means the proliferation of electronic devices with screens, as well as energy-efficient lighting, is increasing exposure to blue wavelengths, especially after sundown. If you must use a computer at night I encourage you to download the software **f.lux** http://justgetflux.com/) onto your computer. It is safe and lowers the levels of blue light on your computer after the sun goes down.

Read a book or listen to soothing music. You can before going to bed (preferably in another room, not you bedroom), but it is best to turn off the light and put the book down when you feel tired before going to sleep. Practice deep breathing to relax before you go to sleep. Keep the room dark whenever possible. The bedroom should be dark and devoid of any light whatsoever so that your brain can correctly interpret sleep cues throughout the night. When you wake up in the morning, try to get some sunlight. It is also recommended that you sleep in a room where the temperature is between 60-68 degrees fahrenheit.

Diet (see Appendix 8)

A healthy diet makes neurofeedback more effective. Try to minimize processed foods at home and fast foods while on the run. White sugar, artificial sweeteners, saturated fats, simple carbohydrates, and excess salt in your diet should be avoided. These directly affect the brain and create cravings for these items.

Refined carbohydrates should be eliminated from the diet of most individuals. For those who suffer from mood swings or depression (not to mention hyperactivity or hypoglycemia), overuse of sweeteners in general has been implicated as a contributor. Try to reduce or eliminate the use of stimulant beverages (coffee, coke, and other caffeinated soft drinks), and reduce or eliminate the use of alcoholic beverages. Whenever possible, eliminate all food dyes and food preservatives from the diet. It is recommended to eliminate fats/oils including "palm oil" which is a ... for a hydrogenation process.

... nce to support most "fad" diets. The diet ... ...esearch that is supported by the majority of health professionals is the Mediterranean Diet. The Paleo Diet and Ketogenic Diet are also receiving positive medical reviews. The Mediterranean Diet is a diet that supports heart and brain health while reducing the risk of cancer, and a variety of inflammatory diseases. A well-balanced diet of fruits, nuts, vegetables, whole grains, and fish and lean meat proteins are important. Try to avoid eating after 8:00 pm; or two hours before bedtime.

Practice Diaphragmatic Breathing (see Appendix 9)

Using this breathing during the day and during your neurofeedback sessions will help enhance the benefits of neurofeedback. How often should I practice this exercise? At first, practice this exercise 5–10 minutes about 3–4 times per day. Gradually increase the amount of time you spend doing this exercise, and perhaps even increase the effort of the exercise by placing a book on your abdomen.

Counseling

If you have a history of trauma in your background, or have experienced anxiety, depression, or other mental health disorder, it is important to consider having a counselor or therapist you can go to and work with to enhance your overall mental health.

Appendix 1

Client Bill of Rights and Responsibilities Regarding Biofeedback and Neurofeedback

Below is a sample of a Client/Patient Bill of Rights and Responsibilities form, which you might be asked to sign.

We want to encourage you, as a client of (Business Name), to speak openly with your clinical provider, take part in your assessment and treatment choices, and promote your own safety and well-being by being well informed and involved in your biofeedback (BFB) and neurofeedback (NFB) treatment services. You are encouraged to think of yourself as a partner in your care, and therefore to know your rights as well as your responsibilities during your course of treatment. (Business Name) provides various educational interventions, assessment protocols, and treatment services, a few of which are still considered, by some, to be experimental.

Client Rights:

- You have the right to receive considerate, respectful and compassionate treatment in a safe setting, free from all forms of abuse, neglect, or mistreatment, regardless of your age, gender, race, national origin, religion, sexual orientation, gender identity or disabilities. You have the right to inquire about and discuss ethical issues related to your care at all times, and to voice your concerns about the care you receive.

- You have the right to be told by your treatment provider about your diagnosis and possible prognosis, the benefits and risks of treatment, and the expected outcome of treatment. You have the right to give written informed consent before any non-emergency procedure begins, and to understand the costs of assessment and treatment before you begin.

- You, your family, and friends with your permission, have the right to participate in decisions about your treatment, including the right to refuse/withdraw from treatment.

- You have the right to decide not to receive BFB/NFB treatment from us. If you wish, we can provide you with the names of other qualified BFB/NFB providers.

- You have the right to ask questions about protocol and procedures used during all BFB/NFB sessions, and to ask questions about NFB/BFB techniques and to prevent the use of certain training techniques if you feel unsure of them, and to participate in setting goals and evaluating progress towards meeting them.

- You have the right to have all that you say treated confidentially and be informed of state law placing limitations on confidentiality in the NFB/BFB relationship. Under certain circumstances, we are required by law to reveal information obtained during NFB/BFB to other persons or agencies without your permission. Also, we are not required to inform you of our actions in this regard. These situations are as follows: (a) if you threaten bodily harm or death to yourself or another person, we are required by law to notify the victim and appropriate law enforcement agencies; (b) if a court of law issues a subpoena; (c) if you are in NFB/BFB training or being tested by a court of law, the results of the treatment or tests must be revealed to the court; (d) if you have given us information concerning non-accidental injury and neglect to minors or incompetent adults; or (e) if you are in the process of filing a workman's compensation claim or file such in the future.

Client Responsibilities—You Are Expected to:

1. Provide complete and accurate information, including your full name, address, home telephone number, date of birth, and employer when it is required.
2. Provide complete and accurate information about your health and medical history, including present condition, past illnesses, hospital stays, medicines, vitamins, herbal products, and any other matters that pertain to your health, including perceived safety risks.
3. Ask questions when you do not understand information or instructions. If you believe you cannot follow through with your treatment plan, you are responsible for telling your treatment provider. You are responsible for outcomes if you do not follow the treatment plan.

4. Provide complete and accurate information about your finances and to pay your fees in accordance with the arrangement you pre-established with (Business Name).
5. Set and keep appointments with your provider, and be on time for your appointments. **Appointments cancelled without at least 24-hour notice are subject to a $50 charge.**
6. Help plan your therapy goals, and keep your NFB/BFB provider informed of your progress toward meeting your goals.
7. Inform your NFB/BFB provider of any problems you have which may influence your progress or which may be potentially harmful to yourself or others.
8. Notify (Business Name) if you intend to discontinue training.

I have read and understand my rights.

Appendix 2

Informed Consent

Below is a sample of an Informed Consent form you might be asked to sign.

The purpose of this form is to obtain your voluntary consent to participate in one or more methods of quantitative electroencephalography (QEEG) brain mapping, peripheral biofeedback, neurofeedback, other forms of relaxation and stress reduction interventions, and to disclose potential benefits and risks associated with these interventions. (Business Name) provides various educational interventions, assessment protocols, and health care services, a few of which are still considered, by some, to be experimental.

QEEG Brain Mapping

To determine an appropriate neurofeedback training plan, a QEEG performed by (Business Name) using the (Company) expert referential database system will be conducted.

(Business Name) will assess your need for having a QEEG. To engage in neurofeedback, you will be required to have a QEEG assessment. In other instances, to help verify a disorder, your doctor, or another health care professional, may recommend you have a QEEG. A QEEG consists of placing a cap on your head with 20 electrodes/sensors. Each site will be cleansed, and a special gel will be placed under each sensor to insure proper conductivity to read your brainwaves. Preparation and the assessment procedure take approximately 1 hour.

Benefits: QEEG may help me further understand and/or confirm the problems/symptoms, disorders, and/or diagnosis for which I am seeking assessment and health care services.

Side Effects/Risks: QEEG may result in my feeling anxious/apprehensive, and/or uncomfortable during the procedure, and sad/disappointed regarding findings from the procedure. The cap may cause you to have a mild headache.

Forensic Services: QEEG brain mapping for purposes of neurofeedback is not a medical procedure and is not done at (Business Name) for purposes of medical diagnosis. Data collected is not done in a manner that meets the Daubert criteria for admissibility of evidence in court. (Business Name) does not provide forensic services or diagnosis for TBI. We do not accept invitations for depositions. Those seeking a diagnosis for TBI or any other medical or mental disorder should seek services of a medical physician or a forensic neuropsychologist. Your signature below indicates you agree not to request or seek such services from us presently or in the future, or through third parties such as legal counsel or insurance companies.

Client/Patient Rights. You have the right to:

- Decide not to receive QEEG brain mapping services from us. If you wish, we can provide you with the names of other qualified QEEG providers.
- End the QEEG at any time.
- Ask questions about protocol and procedures used during the QEEG procedure, and to ask questions about QEEG techniques if you feel unsure of them.
- Have all that you say treated confidentially and be informed of state law placing limitations on confidentiality in the QEEG relationship. Under certain circumstances, we are required by law to reveal information obtained during a QEEG assessment to other persons or agencies without your permission. Also, we are not required to inform you of our actions in this regard. These situations are as follows: (a) if you threaten bodily harm or death to yourself or another person, we are required by law to notify the victim and appropriate law enforcement agencies; (b) if a court of law issues a subpoena; (c) if you are having a QEEG or being tested by a court of law, the results of the QEEG assessment must be revealed to the court; (d) if you have given us information concerning non-accidental injury and neglect to minors or incompetent adults; or (e) if you are in the process of filing a workman's compensation claim or file such in the future.

Equipment/Software: QEEG measures will involve the use of the. (Business Name) software and hardware (equipment type). (Business Name) products are FDA registered. QEEG maps are produced using (report system).

Neurofeedback Training

Neurofeedback involves several electrodes/sensors being placed on the scalp and earlobes. The sensors detect brain wave activity including alpha, beta, delta, and theta brainwaves. Individual brainwaves are measured and displayed on a computer screen revealing your brainwave activity. Through instruction you can learn to train down or train up certain brainwaves associated with stress management, attentional, cognitive and/or emotional deficits and related disorders. In some cases, neurofeedback must be considered as experimental. Treatments last from 10–30 minutes and may occur two or more times per week for an average of 30–40, and in some cases more than 40 sessions.

Benefits: Neurofeedback (NFB) is known to assist individuals by decreasing symptoms associated with brain and central nervous system dysfunction. Other benefits include the possibility of reducing problem behaviors and increasing peak performance. In many cases, neurofeedback is experimental when used to a treat certain disorders. Please feel free to ask for a more detailed explanation regarding your problem area or treatment interest.

Side Effects/Risks: Neurofeedback will not interfere with most other treatments. Neurofeedback has few side effects when administered properly. The most common side effects of neurofeedback include improved sleep, more awareness of dreams, feeling calmer, feeling more energy, and feeling more focused. Temporary side effects such as headaches, insomnia, anxiety, feeling giddy, agitated, or irritated may occur during or right after a neurofeedback session.

However, these side effects can be adjusted and eliminated immediately in most cases. It is also possible that you might fall asleep during or after neurofeedback sessions.

Client Rights. You have the right to:

- Decide not to receive neurofeedback services from us. If you wish, we can provide you with the names of other qualified neurofeedback providers.
- End neurofeedback sessions at any time.
- Ask questions about protocol and procedures used during neurofeedback training, and to ask questions about techniques if you feel unsure of them.
- Have all that you say treated confidentially and be informed of state law placing limitations on confidentiality in the neurofeedback relationship. Under certain circumstances, we are required by law to reveal information obtained during training to other persons or agencies without your permission. Also, we are not required to inform you of our actions in this regard. These situations are as follows: (a) if you threaten bodily harm or death to yourself or another person, we are required by law to notify the victim and appropriate law enforcement agencies; (b) if a court of law issues a subpoena; (c) if you are being treated with neurofeedback, at the direction of an attorney or medical doctor for legal purposes, the results of the training or tests must be revealed to the court; (d) if you have given us information concerning non-accidental injury and neglect to minors or incompetent adults;

or (e) if you are in the process of filing a workman's compensation claim or file such in the future.

Equipment/Software: Neurofeedback treatment will involve the use of the (Business Name) software and hardware (equipment type). (Business Name) products are FDA registered.

Other Methods: Other treatment methods may not work as rapidly as the methods and modalities described above. Alternative methods of treatment and/or therapy include traditional medical treatments, medications, the use of supplements, the use of relaxation techniques, group and individual therapy.

Choosing the Right Intervention: The interventions described above are voluntary, *not* mandatory. You will not be pressured for not participating. You may withdraw from/ stop receiving neurofeedback training sessions at any time without consequence.

Consent

I voluntarily consent to participate in and undergo the assessment and/or intervention methods and modalities described above. I understand that I am free to withdraw my consent and to discontinue participation in the interventions/ modalities/methods described above at any time. The natural consequences and potential risks and benefits have been fully explained to me by (Business Name).

Permission

My signature below indicates that I have read, reviewed and understand this informed consent (and/or I have had the form and its contents read to me and explained to me), and I consent to participate in the procedures described above. I understand I may ask questions at any time, and may request to stop interventions at any time.

I have read and understand my rights.

Appendix 3

Financial Policy

Below is a sample of a Financial Policy you might be asked to sign.

The following information offers some guidelines regarding our financial policy.

- We do not take health insurance and are not a Medicaid/Medicare provider.
- **Please be prepared to pay for services at the time services are rendered.**
- Please be aware that **you are ultimately responsible for the timely payment of your account**.
- A $35.00 bank fee will be charged for any returned checks.
- Past due accounts of 90 days or more may be subject to collections.
- Except in cases of emergencies, **we require a minimum 24-hour notice if you cannot keep your scheduled appointment**. We reserve the right to charge for appointments canceled or broken without

a 24-hour notice. Our fee for missed appointments (those without a 24-hour cancellation) is $50.00 per session hour.

- For your convenience, we accept cash, personal check, MasterCard, Visa, Discover Card and American Express.

If you have any questions regarding our policy, please feel free to ask us. We are here to help you!

I have read and agree to the conditions as outlined:

Appendix 4

Authorization for Release of Information (HIPAA)

Below is a sample of an Authorization for Release of Information form you might be asked to sign.

Name: **Date of Birth:**   **Client:**

(Business Name) is authorized to release protected health information about the above-named individual to the entities named below. The purpose is to inform the professionals or persons listed below in keeping with the patient's instructions.

Entity to Receive Information Check each person/entity that you approve to receive information	**Description of information to be released.** Check each that can be given to the person/ entity on the left in the same section.
☐ Voice Mail	☐ Results of QEEG /Assessments ☐ NFB Treatment Sessions ☐ Other
☐ Spouse (provide name & phone number)	☐ Results of QEEG /Assessments ☐ NFB Treatment Sessions ☐ Other

☐ Parent (provide name & phone number)	☐ Results of QEEG /Assessments ☐ NFB Treatment Sessions ☐ Other
☐ Other (provide name & phone number)	☐ Results of QEEG /Assessments ☐ NFB Treatment Sessions ☐ Other
☐ Your E-mail:	☐ Results of QEEG /Assessments ☐ NFB Treatment Sessions ☐ Other
☐ Other E-mail: Name of Person E-mail will go to:	☐ Results of QEEG /Assessments ☐ NFB Treatment Sessions ☐ Other

Personal Information: I understand that I have the right to revoke this authorization at any time and that I have the right to inspect or copy the protected health information to be disclosed as described in this document. I understand that a revocation is not effective in cases where the information has already been disclosed but will be effective going forward.

I understand that information used or disclosed because of this authorization may be subject to redisclosure by the recipient and may no longer be protected by federal or state law.

I understand that I have the right to refuse to sign this authorization and that my treatment will not be conditioned on signing. This authorization shall be in effect until revoked by the individual named above.

_____   _____

Signature of Person or Personal Representative   Date

Description of Personal Representative's Authority (attach necessary documentation)

Appendix 5

Client Acknowledgements

Below is a sample of a Client Acknowledgement form you might be asked to sign.

Benefits of Neurofeedback

The FDA recognizes that all interventions pose risks and benefits. Typically, the benefits of neurofeedback far outweigh the risks and although on occasion, it can result in non-serious adverse events. As a form of biofeedback it falls under the category of other low risk activities such as progressive relaxation, hypnosis, breathing exercises meditation, yoga and massage. The benefits are usually experienced as improved focus, enhanced concentration, increased energy, higher quality sleep, decreased moodiness, diminished agitation, and reduction in anxiety as well as reductions in other physical symptoms typically related to stress such as headache.

Risks of Neurofeedback

Training with neurofeedback can occasionally result in adverse response(s) that temporarily increases symptoms that are typically associated with relaxation and calming of the central nervous system such as fatigue, headaches, lightheadedness, dizziness, irritability, moodiness, weeping, insomnia, agitation, and difficulties with focus and anxiety. These reactions, if they occur, are temporary and typically only last 24–48 hours. Once clients/patients become more relaxed and aware, they tend to integrate past emotional issues and these symptoms subside.

I have participated in a QEEG brain map, have read the notations above, and I would like to pursue neurofeedback training. I understand that:

1. NFB is not a quick fix or cure all but reduces symptom severity over time through training to improved central nervous system (CNS) regulation.
2. The average number of NFB sessions to achieve enduring change is 40 sessions.
3. On average, most people require 15 sessions to experience symptom changes. If symptom changes do not occur within 15–20 sessions it is most likely due to either metabolic or life stress issues.
4. Side effects may result from prescribed drugs when dosage is not reduced over sessions.
5. Some agitation or irritability may occur for a couple of weeks following the 15th session.
6. The chronic use of psychotropic drugs impedes progress.
7. Reducing dependence on pharmaceuticals is a key objective of the training program.
8. That client must make efforts to manage diet, exercise, sleep and stressful activities to achieve the best results.

9. Failure to work with clinicians to make lifestyle changes can reduce or mitigate effects of NFB training.
10. Hair analysis or organic acid tests will be required if progress is slow.
11. Clients are expected to complete weekly progress reports the day before their NFB Training sessions. Completion of weekly progress reports helps guide us in providing the best quality of care.

I have read and understand the items outlined above:

Appendix 6

QEEG Brain Mapping Preparation Checklist

Below is a sample of a QEEG Preparation Checklist you might be given.

The following instructions are for the patient to review and follow before they come in for a QEEG, and will help assure that the best results possible are acquired. **PLEASE PAY ATTENTION to bolded print.**

1. Illness. If you are sick, call to reschedule even if you only have a cold.

2. Sleep. You should get a good night's sleep before the QEEG (let us know if you have any sleep problems or disturbances).

3. Hair and Scalp. Your hair needs to be clean and dry. Use a pH neutral detergent shampoo such as Neutrogena Anti-Residue or Suave Clarifying shampoo the night before or the on the day of your scheduled appointment. Wash your hair three times. If you have a hair weaves, toupee, or corn-rows, please remove them (if they are removeable), before your appointment. **No chemical treatments may be administered (coloring, perms, relaxers, etc.) within 48 hours before the QEEG. DO NOT use oils, lotions, mousse, gels, or hairsprays. Hair must be free of beads, weaves, etc. Make sure your hair is completely dry before coming for the QEEG.**

Please bring a comb or brush.

4. Medications. The QEEG assessment is often cleaner and easier to read if there are no medications in the brain. If the client is taking stimulant medication (i.e., ADHD medication), it is preferable to do the QEEG recording after the patient has stopped taking the medication for *up to 48* hours prior. **The client MUST check with his/ her prescribing physician or health care provider to determine if it is possible to stop taking the stimulants 48 hours prior to the QEEG. If 48 hours is not advisable 12–24 is the next preferred length of time. Do not make changes in any other medication(s) unless authorized by your physician. If you are taking medications for anxiety, depression, or sleep please do NOT stop taking these medications without first consulting with your prescriber. If you prescriber approves, please bring these medications with you the day of your QEEG and take them after the QEEG assessment has been conducted.**

5. Over the Counter Medications and Supplements. ***Unless prescribed by a physician or licensed health care provider***, client should avoid taking any over the counter medication or supplements for 2 or 3 days prior to the QEEG. This includes medications and supplements such as such as:

acetaminophen (Tylenol), Advil (Motrin/ibuprofen), aspirin, analgesics, antihistamines/allergy medications (Benadryl, Claritin, Allegra, Zyrtec), cough and cold medicines, herbs, nasal sprays, nutraceuticals (sports drinks, Gator Aid, etc.), food **supplements (including amino acids), vitamins, or other similar products).** If you have any questions about these items, please contact your QEEG clinician.

6. Caffeinated Beverages. The client should *NOT* drink excessive amounts of coffee, tea, or caffeinated beverages in the morning of the testing (i.e., one cup is fine) and the patient should *NOT* drink soft drinks with excessive amounts of caffeine in them, i.e., Red Bull, highly caffeinated soft drinks, for at least 15 hours prior to the QEEG.

7. Alcohol and Drugs. Alcohol should be avoided 24 hours prior to your session. Marijuana should be avoided 24–72 hours prior to your session.

8. Contact Lenses. Portions of the QEEG require that your eyes be closed for up to 15 minutes. If you wear contact lenses, please be prepared to remove them if they create discomfort with your eyes closed.

9. Please bring a complete list of medications you take on a daily or regular basis with you when you come for your QEEG.

The day of the QEEG, the client should:

1. Eat a high protein breakfast.

2. **Women should not wear any makeup on the forehead or ear lobes**.

3. Drink plenty of water the day before the QEEG recording.

4. Use the restroom to prior to the start of the QEEG.

5. **No jewelry on neck or ears**.

6. **Nicotine should be avoided 3 hours prior to your session.**

7. **Bring any medications or supplements you would like to take after your QEEG is complete.**

On the day of your QEEG brain map appointment, plan to spend a minimum of 90 minutes in the office. In addition, you will likely need several minutes to fix your hair following your appointment. Facilities are provided.

PLEASE NOTE: Lack of sleep, medications, low blood sugar, and movement of the eyes, tongue, head or body, may affect the results.

Appendix 7

Sleep Hygiene

The following guidelines are a summary of what constitutes good sleep hygiene.

Maintain a bedtime routine (wake and sleep pattern) seven days a week, and establish a regular relaxing sleep routine. Make sure your bedroom is comfortable and relaxing. High quality mattress and pillows are important. Try to avoid emotionally upsetting conversations and activities before trying to go to sleep. Don't dwell on or bring your problems, or the problems of others, to bed. Associate your bed with sleep. It's not a good idea to use your bed to watch TV, listen to the radio, or read.

I advise patients/clients that getting less than 6.5 /7 hours of sleep each night leaves you cognitively impaired. When a person doesn't sleep well, nothing in the human body works well. Sleep deprivation can result in both physical and mental health problems including but not limited to obesity, diabetes, cardiovascular disease, Alzheimer's, cancer, depression, anxiety disorders and attentional and cognitive functioning deficits and disorders.

Some general guidelines include:

- Do not eat before going to sleep and avoid eating big meals before bedtime.
- Eliminate stimulants such as caffeine, nicotine, and alcohol too close to bedtime.
- Go outside and get 30-60 minutes of daylight / natural light every day. Daytime light exposure helps you maintain a healthy circadian rhythm.
- Exercise daily or minimally 3-4 times per week. Exercise promotes good sleep.
- Try to avoid napping during the day.

What can Cause Sleep Problems / Disturbances?

Sleep hygiene is important for everyone from childhood through adulthood, and promotes healthy sleep, while minimizing sleep problems and disorders. Sleep problems and disturbances include but are not limited to:

- Going to bed late.
- Taking too long to fall asleep.
- Waking up frequently during the night.
- Waking up feeling tired and feeling like you need more sleep.

Sleep problems like those listed above can occur for many reasons including:

- A sleep partner who snores.
- Animals sleeping on your bed.
- Excessive light in your bedroom.

- Eating or drinking stimulants, i.e., caffeine beverages, chocolate, etc.
- Alcohol
- Certain medications (always check for medication side effects).
- Electro-magnetic Fields (EMFs), i.e., wifi, cellphones, remote controlled and Bluetooth devices.

Blue light from the use of electronic devices including computers, phones, tablets, nooks, etc., before going to bed. Ways to minimize blue light include:

- Turning down the brightness level on your device
- Put your devices away 1-2 2 hours before bedtime
- Use apps that allow you to change your device's traditional blue light screen to a healthier red or yellow light. Some apps and programs for reducing blue light include Twilight, NeyetLight; F.lux; and Lux.
- Wear amber-tinted sunglasses while using your device at night.

Unfortunately, most people spend their days indoors, do not get enough bright daylight, and then spend their evenings in bright artificial light, i.e., florescent and LED lighting. This results in your body clock/circadian rhythm getting out of cycle with the natural rhythm of daylight and nighttime darkness.

What are The Consequences of Poor Sleep?

Poor sleep impacts many aspects of your mental and physical health. Some of the negative impacts include:

- You reaction time slows down.
- Your cognition functioning including attention, focus, and concentration are impacted.
- Memory worsens and learning deficits occur.
- Emotions can become poorly regulated. One can become overly emotional or your emotions become muted. Irritability and anger can become more problematic. Anxiety and or depression can worsen.
- Immune function and health deteriorates including high blood pressure.

People Need an Average of Eight Hours of Sleep per Night

There are numerous studies that have looked into the quality of sleep and how people are affected when they have poor sleep or not enough sleep. The majority of research suggests that people need between 7.5 and 9.5 hours of sleep per night.

If you are not sure about how much sleep you are getting there are various sleep tracking devices such as *Fit Bit® Oura Ring®* and *S+ ResMed®* that will keep track of your sleep and sleep quality.

Appendix 8

Diet

There is no science to support most "fad" diets. The diet with the most research that is supported by most of health professionals is the Mediterranean diet; and the Paleo and Ketogenic diets continue to gain support by various health care professionals. These diets support heart and brain health while reducing the risk of cancer, and a variety of inflammatory diseases. A well-balanced diet of fruits, nuts, vegetables, whole grains, and fish and lean meat proteins are important. Try to avoid eating after 8:00 pm at night.

There are numerous articles and health care professionals who encourage people to eat organic whenever possible and some of the best foods, herbs, and spices for body and brain health include:

• Avocado • Berries • Broccoli • Celery • Citrus • Dark Chocolate (70% + cocoa) • Grapes

• Green tea • Oatmeal • Onions • Oranges • Oregano • Parsley • Red Peppers • Sage

ke supplements that they do not
much good. Many supplements
DA and there is no guarantee
fore taking supplements check
lt with a registered dietician/
nutritionist. Good quality and proper dosage are important
if you are going to use them (i.e., not all fish oils/omega-3s are
the same). When needed, patients should consider taking a
multi-vitamin/mineral supplement, Omega-3 Fish oils, CQ-
10, probiotics, and a good digestive enzyme. Patients should
always check with their physician or a qualified nutritionist
or dietician first before taking any supplements.

Recommended Reading

Amen, D. G. (2005). *Making a good brain great.* New York: Three Rivers Press.

Amen, D. G. (1998). *Change your brain, change your life: The breakthrough program for conquering anxiety, depression, obsessiveness, anger and impulsiveness.* New York: Three Rivers Press.

Begley, S. (2007). *Train your mind, change your brain: How a new science reveals our extraordinary potential to transform ourselves.* New York: Ballentine Books.

Kotulak, R. (1996). *Inside the brain: Revolutionary discoveries of how the mind works.* Kansas City, MO: Andrews McMeel Publishing.

Moyers, B. (1993). *Healing and the mind.* New York: Doubleday.

Robbins, Jim. (2000). *A symphony in the brain.* New York: Grove Hills.

CPSIA information can be obtained
at www.ICGtesting.com
Printed in the USA
BVHW042131210120
570100BV00010B/147